Atkins Diet Plan for Beginners

Essential and Only Guide Needed To Getting Started With Atkins Diet

Disclaimer

All rights reserved. No part of this Book may be reproduced, stored in a retrieval system, or transmitted, in any form, or by any means, including mechanical or electronic, without the prior written permission of the author, nor be otherwise circulated in any form.

While the author has made every effort to ensure that the ideas, guidelines and information presented in this Book are safe, they should be used at the reader's discretion. The author cannot be held responsible for any personal or commercial damage arising from the application or misinterpretation of information presented herein.

Table of Contents

Introduction 4

Chapter 1 – The Atkins Diet Program Basics 6

Chapter 2 – The Induction Phase of the Atkins Diet Program 14

Chapter 4 - The Balancing Phase of the Atkins Diet Program 36

Chapter 5 - Other Things you Need to Know About the Balancing Phase 42

Chapter 6 - The Pre-Maintenance Phase of the Atkins Diet Program 48

Chapter 7 - The Lifetime Maintenance Phase of the Atkins Diet Program 56

Chapter 8 – Frequently Asked Questions about the Atkins Diet Program 62

Conclusion

Introduction

I want to thank you and congratulate you for purchasing the book, *"Atkins Diet Plan for Beginners - Essential and Only Guide Needed to Getting Started with Atkins Diet"*.

This book contains proven steps and strategies on how to get started losing weight through the Atkins Diet Program. Let this book be your guide to successful weight loss. It lays down all the necessary information to get you through from one phase to another. The information in this book should help you every step of the way of the Atkins Diet Program.

Included in this book are guidelines for starting from the Induction Phase to the next three phases of the program. You have a detailed list of acceptable foods from each phase. This book also provides you with serving size suggestions and the corresponding net carb content for the acceptable foods. You also have a few examples of menu.

Through this book, you will learn about all the things you need to expect during the program including side effects and the different ways to deal with them. All you need is this book to start losing weight successfully and permanently through the Atkins diet.

Thanks again for purchasing this book, I hope you enjoy it!

Chapter 1 – The Atkins Diet Program Basics

Since the 1970s, people thought that the best way to shake off excess pounds is by counting calories and fat grams. Today, however, we are well aware of better and easier ways.

Chances are this is not your first encounter with Atkins Diet. It has become one of the most popular and widely relied on diet plan for people who want to lose weight fast without exerting much effort to physical exercise.

Invented by Dr. Robert Atkins, this diet plan does not involve counting calories. It is not concerned with fat grams either. Rather, it focuses on carbohydrate consumption.

How does this diet plan work?

To understand how this diet plan works, you must first familiarize yourself with the way body creates energy. There are two major sources of energy: fat and glucose.

There is a widespread misconception about fat. Most people obsess about restricting their diet to low fat foods. They feel that such will make them slimmer or at least prevent unwanted weight gain. Reducing fat consumption is essential. However, you must make it a point to get enough. Otherwise, the only way to get sufficient energy is to turn to carbohydrates.

Carbohydrates are not so bad as fat, right? This is where the danger lies. Do you know what happens to your body when you eat more carbohydrates than your body requires? Excess carbohydrates are converted and stored as fat. You may now be wondering whether it is better to consume less carbs and more fat. That is where the Atkins diet comes in.

Overweight issues usually arise from insulin level and blood sugar problems. As you know, insulin is a hormone that is fat producing. If you work at limiting your consumption of foods that generate excessive insulin release, you are likely to lose unwanted weight. In other words, Atkins diet helps you regulate insulin level, which in turn, works in reducing fat from the body.

The Atkins diet program is widely recognized because of its effectiveness for weight loss. Why? For the simple reason that it is structured in such a way that teaches the body and trains metabolism to burn fat rather than store it. How does this happen?

The body uses both fat and glucose as energy sources, but it uses mostly glucose. When you restrict your carbohydrate consumption, it forces your body to use fat as energy source. This does not mean you have to consume fat heavily. Rather, stored fat are converted to usable energy until fat in specific body areas have been exhausted.

As a result, your body is trained to use entirely fatty acids as its energy source, so you burn fat rather than store it. This results to weight loss. As you reduce your carb consumption, your body enters a metabolic process referred to as ketosis. It is a state of fat burning.

In this diet program, you are encouraged to eliminate starchy carb and sugary foods from your diet. For one, this kind of food is either low or completely lacking in nutrients, and such kind of food includes bagels, cereals and processed foods.

Whole grains and high carb vegetables and fruits may offer nutritional value, but in the Atkins program, you need to regulate your consumption of such foods especially in the initial phase. Instead of high carb foods, you need to consume more leafy greens, protein foods, healthy fat food sources and low carb vegetables.

Four Phases of the Atkins Program

The Atkins diet program consists of different phases. Here is a quick overview of the four phases including what you need to expect from each phase.

Phase One: Induction Phase

The first phase of the diet program is undoubtedly the most limiting. You will probably find it the most challenging of the four phases especially if you are fond of eating high carb foods. The switch is rather difficult. While you are not required to eliminate carbohydrate foods from your diet completely, it is still advisable for you to keep it at a minimum.

Entering the induction phase, you must steer clear from high carb fruits and vegetables. Instead, you can eat low carb vegetables including pepper, mushrooms, alfalfa sprouts and leafy green vegetables. Instead of carb loading, you are encouraged to eat more protein food sources such as meat, eggs and chicken.

You are also advised to consume healthy fats that include olive oil. Cheeses like cheddar, mozzarella and cream cheese are acceptable. You may use herbs and spices such as cilantro, basil and dill among others too.

While this phase is the toughest, it also offers the quickest way to weight loss. The induction phase goes on for a minimum of two weeks. You can continue on this phase until you are 15 pounds away from your weight goal.

Phase Two: Balancing Phase

The goal of the second phase of the Atkins diet program is to help you find your personal carb balance. Some of the foods that you were deprived of during the first phase are allowed in this one. In the second phase, you may add high carb vegetables, whole milk, yogurt, berries, nuts, seeds and other cheeses like cottage cheese in your diet.

You have to stay on this phase until you are only 10 pounds away from your weight goal.

Phase Three: Fine Tuning Phase

This is the phase where you have to reintroduce more carbohydrate food sources. While doing so, you are also expected to reach your weight goal. The third phase allows you to include the following in your diet: whole grains, starchy vegetables, legumes and additional fruits.

Phase Four: Lifetime Maintenance

By the time you reach this phase, you should already be in your ideal weight. While your goal for the first three phases is to lose weight, all that changes in this phase. Your goal at this point is to keep your weight in control. In which case, you should still be mindful of the way you consume carbohydrates. Abandon mindfulness and you are most likely to regain the weight that you have already lost. To make sure you do not over consume carbs, you are encouraged to monitor your weight regularly

There is no due date for this phase. If you want to maintain your shape, you must make a permanent change.

Chapter 2 – The Induction Phase of the Atkins Diet Program

The Induction Phase does not necessarily embody the entire Atkins diet program. It is only first of four phases of the plan. As you have learned from the previous chapter, the first phase is meant to jumpstart your weight loss. Each phase should be able to help you find your body's ideal amount of carb requirement.

The Atkins diet does not encourage you to starve yourself. Rather, it encourages you to find your carb balance. This way, you get sufficient nourishment but at the same time, lose weight. However, why is it important to find your carb balance? Won't you lose weight faster if you just starve your body from carbs?

The problem with that kind of strategy is that hunger spurs appetite. The hungrier you get, the tougher it becomes to control your appetite. However, if you find your carb balance, you can lose weight and at the same time get your much needed nourishment. This way, you remain active and alert. Moreover, carb balance is different from one person to another. In other words, you have to find your own balance.

What is the goal and purpose of the Induction Phase?

The main goal of this phase is to train your body to turn to fat for energy rather than to glucose. A regular diet that is carb loaded requires your body to rely primarily on glucose as its energy source. Therefore, when you reduce your carb consumption, your body makes the necessary adjustment by burning fat rather than carbs for energy. This will kick start the process of weight loss.

In order to reach this goal, you must reduce your Net Carb consumption to 20 grams a day on average. You can reduce it to as low as 18 grams a day but not lower, or 22 grams a day but not any higher. Choose your number according to your personal weight loss goal. However, essentially, at a range of 18 and 22 grams is where most people start to burn fat.

The process wherein the body burns fat is called ketosis. How do you know if your body has reached ketosis? There are ketone-testing strips that you can buy. They test your urine stream and measure the amount of ketones present. You can purchase such strips from your local pharmacy.

If the testing strip indicates any color of pink to purple, you have definitely achieved ketosis. However, for this to be possible, you have to abide by the rules of the Induction phase. Steer clear from sugar, fruits, all breads, all pasta, corn, potato, flour, beans, rice, candy, carrots, milk and everything else that contain more than the daily-recommended carbs.

You have to keep in mind that carbs is present in almost all kinds of food. To make sure you are not duped into taking hidden carbs, it is advisable to get yourself a good quality carb counter. Such will help you stick to your daily **Net Carb** consumption.

What are you allowed to eat during this phase?

Since you are only allowed an average of 20 grams of carbs a day, it makes sense to stick to low carb foods. As mentioned in the overview, you can also eat other foods like protein sources. Below is a list of the acceptable foods during the Induction Phase.

Fish and Other Seafoods

Most fishes and seafoods do not contain carbohydrates. All kinds including sardines, wild salmon, herring, flounder, trout, sole and tuna among many others may be included in your diet.

Crabmeat, clams, squid and shrimp are also acceptable. Oysters and mussels contain carbs, but at a minimum so they are also allowed during this phase. However, you have to be mindful of your portions. Keep your consumption at 4 ounces a day for either mussels or oysters.

Meat and Poultry

You may eat pork, beef, veal, lamb and venison. However, you have to watch out for processed meats. Most are cured with sugar. Remember that the diet program prohibits sugar. Consuming meat cured in sugar will significantly increase your carb count. You can eat some, but when you do, make it a point to include it in your net carb count. Again, it is important to stick to your Net Carb daily recommendation. It is best to avoid processed meat cured by a certain chemical called nitrates.

Fowl is also acceptable during the Induction Phase. This includes chicken, duck, turkey, quail, goose, pheasant, etc.

Eggs

Since eggs are allowed in the Atkins diet, you may as well make it a breakfast staple. There are one hundred ways to cook egg as long as you do not use high carb food items to cook with it. Some of the things you are allowed to add in your egg breakfast include mushrooms, onions, green pepper, feta cheese, basil and oregano.

Cheese

This food item does contain carbohydrate. However, it is okay as long as you do not go over your recommended daily Net Carb consumption. Most cheese contains a gram of carb for every ounce, which means you must limit your consumption to 3 or 4 ounces a day. Some types of cheese contain more carbs than others. For better guideline, you may refer to the list below.

1 ounce Blue Cheese is equivalent to 0.7 gram Net Carbs.

Half a cup Cheddar Cheese is equivalent to 0 gram Net Carbs.

1 ounce Cow Cheese is equivalent to 0.3 gram Net Carbs.

1 ounce Cream Cheese is equivalent to 0.8 gram Net Carbs.

1 ounce Feta Cheese is equivalent to 1.2 grams Net Carbs.

1 ounce Gouda Cheese is equivalent to 0.6 gram Net Carbs.

1 ounce Goat Cheese is equivalent to 0.3 gram Net Carbs.

1 ounce Mozzarella is equivalent to 0.6 gram Net Carbs.

1 tablespoon Parmesan Cheese is equivalent to 0.2 gram Net Carbs.

1 ounce Sheep Cheese is equivalent to 0.3 gram Net Carbs.

1 ounce Swiss Cheese is equivalent to 1.0 gram Net Carbs.

Vegetables

More than 50 percent of your daily net carb consumption must be dedicated to vegetables. To be more specific, you must consume 12 to 15 grams of carbs from vegetables every day. It is then best to prepare meals that include several kinds of vegetables especially those that are low in carbs.

Some of the vegetables with the least carb content include the following.

1 tablespoon Parsley has 0.1 gram Net Carbs.

1 tablespoon Chives has 0.1 gram Net Carbs.

Half a Cup Mushrooms has 1.2 grams Net Carbs.

Half a Cup Jicama has 2.5 grams Net Carbs.

Half a Cup Fennel has 1.8 grams Net Carbs.

Half a Cup Cucumber has 1.0 gram Net Carbs.

Half a Cup Daikon has 1.0 gram Net Carbs.

Half a Cup Endive has 0.4 gram Net Carbs.

Half a Cup Escarol has 0.1 gram Net Carbs.

Half a Cup Raw Alfalfa Sprouts has 0.2 gram Net Carbs.

Half a Cup Raw Chicory greens has 0.1 gram Net Carbs.

Half a Cup Raw Radicchio has 0.7 gram Net Carbs.

Half a Cup Raw Pepper has 2.3 grams Net Carbs.

1 Cup Romaine Lettuce has 0.4 gram Net Carbs.

1 Cup Iceberg Lettuce has 0.2 gram Net Carbs.

1 Cup Raw Arugula has 0.4 gram Net Carbs.

1 Cup Raw Bok Choy has 0.4 gram Net Carbs.

1 Celery stalk has 0.8 gram Net Carbs.

6 Pieces Raw Radishes has 0.5 gram Net Carbs.

Other vegetables have slightly higher carb content. Such includes cabbage, Swiss chard, broccoli, zucchini and cauliflower among others. However, their consumption is still acceptable during the Induction Phase. Your body can benefit from the additional nutrients they provide. However, you have to be mindful about your portions. To get a clearer idea about the net carb content, please refer to this table.

5 pieces Green Olives contains 0.1 gram Net carbs.

5 pieces Black Olives contains 0.7 gram Net carbs.

1 Heart of Palm contains 0.7 gram Net carbs.

Half a cup Raw Broccoli contains 0.8 gram Net carbs.

1 can Artichoke hearts contains 1.0 gram Net carbs.

Half a cup Bamboo Shoots contains 1.2 grams Net carbs.

Half a cup drained Sauerkraut contains 1.2 grams Net carbs.

Half a cup Raw Cauliflower contains 1.4 grams Net carbs.

Half a cup Zucchini contains 1.5 grams Net carbs.

Half a cup Raw Cabbage contains 1.6 grams Net carbs.

Half a cup Unsweetened Rhubarb contains 1.7 grams Net carbs.

Quarter cup Brussels Sprouts contains 1.8 grams Net carbs.

Half a cup Swiss Chard contains 1.8 grams Net carbs.

Half a cup Eggplant contains 2.0 grams Net carbs.

Half a cup Boiled Collard Greens contains 2.0 grams Net carbs.

Quarter cup Boiled Spaghetti Squash contains 2.0 grams Net carbs.

Half a cup Spinach contains 2.2 grams Net carbs.

Quarter cup Kohlrabi contains 2.3 grams Net carbs.

Half a cup Kale contains 2.4 grams Net carbs.

Quarter cup Pumpkin contains 2.4 grams Net carbs.

Half a cup Okra contains 2.4 grams Net carbs.

6 spears Asparagus contain 2.4 grams Net carbs.

Half a cup Raw Summer Squash contains 2.6 grams Net carbs.

Half a cup Turnips contains 3.3 grams Net carbs.

Half a cup Snow peas and snap peas in pod contain 3.4 grams Net carbs.

Half a cup Leeks contains 3.4 grams

Half a cup medium Artichoke contains 3.5 grams Net carbs.

Half a cup Water Chestnuts contains 3.5 grams Net carbs.

Half a cup Raw Avocado contains 3.6 grams Net carbs.

Half a cup Green String Beans contains 4.1 grams Net carbs.

Quarter cup Tomato contains 4.3 grams Net carbs.

Quarter cup Onion contains 4.3 grams Net carbs.

You can do a lot with this selection of vegetables. For green salads, you can add hardboiled eggs or grated cheese of your choice. For additional garnishing, you may also use bacon as much as three slices, which is equal to zero net carb. How is it possible? Aren't bacons supposed to be cured with sugar or maple? Bacons do contain sugar, but the residual sugar is burned because of the cooking process. Suffice to say, you may feel free to garnish your salad with bacon.

Sautéed mushrooms and sour cream may also do. One half cup of sautéed mushrooms contains 1.0-gram net carbs while one tablespoon of sour cream has 0.6 gram of net carbs, so it is completely fine.

Salad dressing of your choice should be no more than 2 grams of net carbs. Two tablespoons of ranch dressing contain 1.4 grams; Caesar dressing contains no more than 0.5 grams while oil and vinegar only have 1.0 grams net carb. You may use lemon, lime juice and blue cheese in moderation as two tablespoons are equivalent to 2.8 and 2.8 grams respectively. You should be especially careful with Italian dressing as two tablespoons contain 3.0 grams net carbs.

Herbs and Spices

As mentioned in the overview, herbs and spices are also acceptable. You can use cayenne pepper, basil, dill, cilantro, sage, oregano, rosemary and tarragon liberally. One tablespoon of each of these herbs and spices contains zero net carb. Ginger and garlic may also be used. However, be reminded that a clove of garlic is equivalent to 0.9 gram net carbs while a tablespoon of ginger is equivalent to 0.8 gram of net carbs.

Fats and Oils

Due to their zero carb content, both fats and oils are acceptable. Nevertheless, you should keep your consumption at a bare minimum. Keep it limited to one tablespoon a day. Another important reminder: when you use oil for cooking your meals, make sure that it does not heat over high temperatures.

Use olive oil for sautéing only. Walnut and sesame oils, on the other hand, must only be used for dressing your salad. For cooking, use canola, grape seed, soybean, walnut, sunflower, safflower and sesame oils. When buying oil, prefer cold pressed or expeller pressed ones. As for fats, you may include mayonnaise and butter in your diet.

Beverage

Drinking enough water will not only keep ill effects of the transition in your diet. It will also help further with weight loss and contribute to your overall health. Make sure to drink eight glasses of eight ounces each of water every day. You can have tap, mineral, spring or filtered water.

Other acceptable beverages for the Induction phase are clear broth, flavored seltzer, unsweetened soy and almond milk including heavy or light cream. Lime and lemon juice are also acceptable as long as you do not drink more than three tablespoons a day.

Chapter 3 - Other Things You Need to Know About the Induction Phase

The recommended number of weeks to spend for the Induction Phase is two weeks at a minimum. However, some people may take longer while others quicker. In fact, some people may not need to go through it at all. It essentially depends on how much weight you want to lose to attain your ideal weight goal.

If your goal is to lose 15 pounds or less, you can jump to the second phase and skip this one altogether. However, if you want to lose more than that, you have to stay on this phase until you are only 15 pounds away from your desired weight. If you want to lose weight fast, you can stay on this phase for three, four or even five weeks.

How does a normal menu on the Atkins Induction Phase look like?

Again, you must consume an average of 20 grams of Net Carbs a day during the first phase. You have been provided with a list of acceptable foods from the previous chapter. You can use that reference to design your diet menu. Just be mindful of the serving size and the corresponding net carbs. Here are a few samples to give you an idea.

Day One

Breakfast: Egg omelet with 3 slices of bacon and 1-ounce cheese of your choice

Lunch: Strips of broiled chicken with Caesar salad minus the croutons

Snack: Diet jello

Dinner: Steak with one serving of green beans

Day Two

Breakfast: Fried egg with 1 slice of American cheese

Lunch: Tuna Salad Wrap

Snack: String Cheese

Dinner: 1 cup of yellow and green beans with grilled chicken

Day Three

Breakfast: Egg and bacon with 3 slices of tomato

Lunch: Cheeseburger patty with green salad

Snack: Deviled Eggs

Dinner: Chicken strips sautéed in olive oil with bacon bits and green beans

What are the side effects?

Because of restricting your carbohydrate consumption to such a low amount compared to what you are used to, you should expect some side effects. Such side effect is referred to as the Atkins induction flu. Atkins dieters commonly experience it. Among the common symptoms are weakness, fatigue, headaches, dizziness, nausea and irritability.

There are two main causes of the Atkins Induction flu. One is carbohydrate withdrawal. Most individuals have a diet that contains 50 percent carbohydrates. The Induction phase forces dieters to cut back to a meager 5 to 10 percent. The huge dietary change results to flu-like symptoms.

To lessen the effects of carb withdrawal or reduce its severity, it is advisable to take vitamin supplements. Take a good multivitamin. It is also recommended to take potassium and calcium supplements.

Another cause of the Atkins Induction flu is dehydration. Diets consisting of low carb foods are usually diuretic. While this is helpful in eliminating unwanted excess water in the body thereby resulting to weight loss, such can also lead to dehydration.

This is why it is important for Atkins dieters to replenish flushed out electrolytes and fluids properly. Otherwise, they will become dehydrated and are likely to suffer the other ill effects that come with it. It is also helpful to take 2 cups of broth every day or half a teaspoon of salt or even 2 tablespoons of soy sauce. That will help replenish lost electrolytes from your body. If your doctor has previously advised you to control your sodium intake, you may consult for further recommendation.

Some dieters start experiencing the side effects 12 hours after cutting back in their carb consumption. However, they usually fade away in a matter of four to five days. For some dieters, however, it may take longer usually as long as an entire week.

Some dieters experience constipation. If you experience such during the Induction Phase, it is advisable to mix 1 tablespoon of psyllium husks with 1 cup of water. Drink this daily. Also, make sure to drink a minimum of eight glasses of water a day. Refer to Chapter 2 for the list of acceptable beverage.

Rules to Live by During the Induction Phase

The number one rule you need to keep in mind during the first phase of your Atkins diet program is that you are only allowed 20 grams on average of net carbs per day. You can go as low as 18 grams or as high as 22 grams, but should never go lower or higher. Most of your carbs should come from low carb vegetables. That means you should get a dose of 3 cups of loosely packed salad a day.

When counting your carbs, count only digestible carbs. Fiber carbs are not included in your 20 grams net carbs daily allowance. That means you should only count carbs that come from sources other than fiber. That is because the body does not digest fiber carbs. In other words, they do not have an impact on your insulin level.

The first phase forbids alcohol, sugar, juice and milk. However, you may use artificial sweeteners that contain sucralose such as Truvia or Splenda. Although their use is permitted, you should always keep it at a minimum.

Start your day with a high protein breakfast. Eat your breakfast within 3 to 4 hours of getting out of bed. Instead of eating bacon and ham every day, try better options like cheese and spinach omelet with diced avocados and fresh salsa toppings. You can also sauté steak strips with bell peppers and onions or get a serving of smoked salmon with cucumber and cream cheese.

Do not wait until you are hungry before you eat lunch. Set a specific time and make sure to eat during that time. Ideally, you need to take lunch four hours after breakfast. An example of an ideal lunch is mixed green with grilled chicken. Tuna salad with fresh avocado is also a good option. You may use commercial dressing for your salad as long as you do not use more than 2 grams of net carbs.

Never skip dinner. It is as important as the first two meals of the day. For dinner, you may have steamed vegetables served with grilled fish. You may also have mashed cauliflower with broiled pork chop. Condiments such as ketchup are not acceptable, but you can always use salt and pepper along with other herbs and spices to make your meals tastier.

Other diets may allow you a cheat day. However, you should not try for one during Induction as such will only compromise the process of ketosis. In other words, you will lose what you have worked so hard for to achieve.

High fat foods such as steak, eggs and bacon are acceptable during this phase. However, that does not mean you have to be liberal in their consumption. Keep in mind that the fat these foods contain can affect caloric content. In which case, it will be wise to keep your consumption of these foods at a minimum. Instead of these high fat foods, you can better rely on lean protein like turkey and chicken breast. You have options so make sure you use them wisely.

Making a change on your diet may be enough to make you lose unwanted weight. If you want to maximize your weight loss during this phase, it is advisable to allot some time for exercise as well. Introduce exercise into your routine. You do not have to do some heavy lifting. Start with simple workouts like walking and other physical activities you enjoy so it will be easier to stick with it once you get started.

Chapter 4 - The Balancing Phase of the Atkins Diet Program

When you are only 15 pounds away from your weight goal, you can move on to the next phase of the Atkins diet program known as the balancing phase. Here, you are presented with a wider variety of food options. In addition to the acceptable foods listed in the Induction Phase, you can now eat nuts, seeds, yogurt, other types of cheese and fruits. However, make sure to reintroduce them into your diet slowly to avoid experiencing further ill effects.

What is the goal and purpose of the Balancing Phase?

The second phase of the Atkins diet program is meant to help you find your personal carb balance for ongoing weight loss. From 20 grams of net carbs in the previous phase, you are now to have a daily allowance of 25 grams of net carbs.

In general, carb balance can range from 30 to 80 grams of net carbs. However, it is not advisable that you reach for the highest immediately. From 20, add 5. With this, you will begin to increase your carb consumption Again, it is advisable to go through the process gradually. Give yourself some time to adjust to the increase of carbs. From there, gradually add more carbs in increments of 5.

Slowly reintroduce more variety in your diet. The second phase is all about finding your balance after all. What does personal carb balance really mean?

There is no set standard carb balance that is applicable to everyone. One's personal carb balance is different from another. Your personal carb balance for instance, is affected by different factors. Your gender, age, activity level and hormonal status, among other factors can affect it. So why is it essential to find that balance?

By definition, personal carb balance is where your body is most suited for continuous weight loss. In other words, if you find your balance, you give your body sufficient energy and at the same time, you put your body at a state of ongoing weight loss.

What are you allowed to eat during this phase?

The list of acceptable foods remains to be restricted but less so as compared in the first phase. The Balancing Phase is more forgiving because it allows you to get your hands on certain foods that were banned from during Induction. You have a broader selection of foods. Again, you must take caution. Make the increase and reintroduction of foods gradual.

In addition to the acceptable foods from Phase 1, you can now consume the following.

Nuts and Seeds

The consumption of higher carb foods into your diet is encouraged. In Phase 2, you can start with nuts and seeds. Slowly increase your carb intake by 5 grams of net carbs a week until you have reached your personal carb balance. Once you have achieved balance, stay there for ongoing weight loss. You can use the list below as reference when computing your carb consumption.

2 tablespoons Hulled Sunflower Seeds is equivalent to 1.1 grams of Net carbs.

7 halves Walnuts is equivalent to 1.5 grams of Net carbs.

10 halves Pecans is equivalent to 1.5 grams of Net carbs.

6 pieces Macadamias is equivalent to 2.0 grams of Net carbs.

5 pieces Brazil Nuts is equivalent to 2.0 grams of Net carbs.

1 ounce Peanuts is equivalent to 2.2 grams of Net carbs.

24 pieces Almonds is equivalent to 2.3 grams of Net carbs.

25 pieces Pistachios is equivalent to 2.5 grams of Net carbs.

9 pieces Cashews is equivalent to 4.4 grams of Net carbs.

Fruits

Now you can enjoy fruits for breakfast or snacks. It is important to take note of their net carb content for each serving size. For instance, quarter a cup of fresh blueberries is equivalent to 4.1 grams of net carbs while the same serving size of honeydew or cantaloupe has 3.5 grams. Quarter a cup of fresh strawberries contain 1.8 grams and the same serving size of fresh raspberries has 1.5 grams of net carbs.

Dairy Products

Some kinds of cheese are acceptable in the first phase. During the Balancing Phase, you will have more options when it comes to dairy products. Here is a list for your reference.

3/4 cup heavy cream has 4.8 grams of net carbs.

Half a cup whole milk has 5.5 grams of net carbs.

Half a cup plain unsweetened yogurt has 5.5 grams of net carbs.

4 ounces tomato juice has 4.2 grams of net carbs.

Quarter a cup lime juice has 5.6 grams of net carbs.

Quarter a cup lemon juice has 5.2 grams of net carbs.

5 ounces mozzarella cheese has 3.0 grams of net carbs.

Half a cup cottage cheese has 4.1 grams of net carbs.

Half a cup ricotta cheese has 3.8 grams of net carbs.

Take advantage of the wider selection in your foods. Keep your meals varied and do not forget to compute your carbs.

Chapter 5 - Other Things you Need to Know About the Balancing Phase

Starting at 25 grams of net carbs, you can increase your carbohydrate consumption at a rate of 5 grams per week. Stop adding only once you have reached your personal carb balance.

How does a normal menu on the Atkins Balancing Phase look like?

With the list of additional acceptable foods in your diet, you should be able to come up with a more varied menu plan. To give you an idea, here is a sample menu plan for the balancing phase.

Day One

Breakfast: Sautéed beef with onions and green bell pepper

Lunch: Grilled Chicken with Caesar salad

Snack: Strawberry Shake

Dinner: Stir fried sesame chicken

Day Two

Breakfast: Creamy eggs and spinach with red bell pepper filling

Lunch: Chicken breast on lettuce with salad greens and shredded Cheese

Snack: A handful of almonds

Dinner: Crustless chicken pot pie with vegetables

Day Three

Breakfast: Cheese and spinach omelet

Lunch: Burger patty with deviled egg and salad greens

Snack: Blueberry yogurt smoothie

Dinner: Ham on romaine with avocado and tomato salad

Rules to Live by During the Balancing Phase

You may be surprised as to how quickly you have lost weight during the Induction Phase. For the second phase, however, you should expect a slower rate of weight loss. It is slow yet steady that is the goal.

As your body learns to adjust from what it had lost during the first phase of the program, you may feel you are no longer losing now. Do not be surprised. The truth is you are still losing. Your body is still working on it so it is best to give it time. Do avoid getting frustrated, average the amount of weight you have lost in a monthly rather than on a weekly basis.

It is also normal to see no difference on the weighing scale as you move to the second phase. You may experience stalls. Prepare yourself for such occurrences. Set proper expectations so you do not get frustrated. When you do, you become less likely to stick with the diet and that will ruin everything you have worked so hard for to achieve.

Understand this. The rate of healthy weight loss is at about 0.5 to 2 pounds a week. You must continue this phase and move on to the third phase once you are 5 to 10 pounds away from your desired weight.

To make sure you achieve successful results, follow these rules.

First, you have to continue what you have started during Induction in terms of consuming low carb vegetables. Eat at least 12 to 15 grams of net carbs coming from foundation vegetables on a daily basis. Just because you have graduated from the initial phase does not mean you can indulge on sugar. It is still unacceptable. Continue to hydrate yourself properly with water or any other acceptable beverages.

Second, do not allow yourself to starve. Allot no more than 3 to 4 hours between meals. Taking snacks is encouraged. Always be mindful of your carb intake and spread out your carb consumption across the day.

Third, avoid getting overexcited about the additional acceptable foods. At best, reintroduce one food group at a time. For instance, for your fist week in the Balancing Phase, add nuts and seeds to your diet to fill in the additional 5-gram net carbs. On your second week, add fruits, etc. If your metabolic rate is slower, do the reintroduction every couple of weeks or whatever works for you.

When you reintroduce one food group to your diet, do it one at a time as well. For instance, add walnuts as snacks today. Before eating almonds, make sure your body has fully adjusted first. You will absolutely know when it feels just right.

Fourth, avoid weighing yourself every day. If you do not see any changes, you may just get frustrated. That may be discouraging and you get more easily tempted to abandon the program. You can choose to measure and weigh in weekly.

Chapter 6 - The Pre-Maintenance Phase of the Atkins Diet Program

By the time you reach the third phase, you are a few stones away from your weight goal. Just like in the balancing phase, it is important to take slow steady steps in increasing your carb consumption here.

What is the goal and purpose of the Pre-Maintenance Phase?

Now, you may have to either continue adding 5 grams a week to your daily carb consumption or by 10 grams. The idea here is to continue finding your personal carb balance so you can lose weight until you have successfully reached your desired weight.

As you go to the process of adding 10-gram additions, you are likely to reach a point where you are no longer losing any more weight. If you reach this point but still has a few more pounds more to lose, take a step back. Drop 10 grams from your daily carb consumption.

Once you have successfully reached your weight goal, focus on preventing any weight gain. To make sure that does not happen, stay at that level of carb intake where you are no longer losing any pounds. Stay on that level for an entire month. If for any reason you start gaining, you simply have to drop 5 or 10 grams from your daily net carb allowance.

The creator of this diet program, Dr. Atkins, recommends that it is best if you lose no more than a single pound a week during this phase. Your body is no longer in ketosis after all. You are allowed to add carbs that have been forbidden in the first two phases. When you do this, you must add back one forbidden carb at a time. The main goal is to prepare the body for the final phase of the program, which is lifetime maintenance.

What are you allowed to eat during this phase?

You have to fine-tune your carb consumption. While you focus on this goal, you need to add more variety in your diet. In addition to the acceptable food list in the first two phases, you are to reintroduce the following into your diet.

Starchy Vegetables

Potatoes, yams, acorn squash and carrots may have been prohibited before. However, in this phase, you can get them back to your menu. As you have learned from the previous phases, it is still important to be wary about your carb consumption. When it comes to the Atkins diet, mindfulness is essential.

So take note that half a portion of potato, baked, contains 10.5 grams net carbs. Baked acorn squash about half a cup is equivalent to 7.8 grams net carbs. And 1 medium carrot has 5.6 grams. Cooked yam of half a portion contains 18.1 grams net carbs.

Legumes

You can fill up your menu with wonderful recipes involving legumes as ingredient. Lentils, navy beans, lima beans and chickpeas among other legumes are now part of your acceptable food list. Here is a list to give you an idea of their net gram content according to serving size.

Quarter cup Kidney Beans is equivalent to 5.8 grams of net carbs.

Half a cup Lentils is equivalent to 12.0 grams of net carbs.

Quarter cup Chickpeas is equivalent to 6.5 grams of net carbs.

Half a cup Black Beans is equivalent to 12.9 grams of net carbs.

Half a cup Pinto Beans is equivalent to 14.6 grams of net carbs.

Quarter cup Great Northern Beans is equivalent to 6.3 grams of net carbs.

Half a cup Navy Beans is equivalent to 18.1 grams of net carbs.

Half a cup Lima Beans is equivalent to 14.2 grams of net carbs.

Grains

After spending a couple of weeks having eggs and yogurt for breakfast, you will be relieved to know that you can have oatmeal or porridge in the Pre-Maintenance Phase. You can also eat brown rice. However, it is still advisable to stick with lower carb grains.

If you will be having brown rice, please take note that half a cup of it contains 20.5 grams of net carbs while one third cup of rolled oats has 19.0 grams. Quarter cup of steel cut oatmeal has the same net carb content.

Additional Fruits

Here's delightful news. You can have more than berries. Apple, banana, red grapes, plum and watermelon are only a few examples of the fruits you can start reintroducing to your diet. Below is a list to help keep your carb counting accurate.

1 small piece Plum has 3.3 grams of net carbs.

Quarter cup Cherries has 4.2 grams of net carbs.

Half a cup Watermelon has 5.2 grams of net carbs.

Half a cup Guava has 5.3 grams of net carbs.

1 small piece Peach has 7.2 grams of net carbs.

Half a piece Red Grapefruit has 7.9 grams of net carbs.

1 piece Kiwi has 8.7 grams of net carbs.

Half a piece Apple has 8.7 grams of net carbs.

Half a cup Mango has 12.5 grams of net carbs.

Half a cup Red Grapes has 13.4 grams of net carbs.

1 small piece Banana has 21.2 grams of net carbs.

Other Things You Need to Know About the Pre-Maintenance Phase

Since you are drawing closer and closer to your desired weight goal, you may start to feel a little more comfortable. You need to bear in mind a couple of things during this phase of the program. Knowing what to expect can save you from frustration.

For one, Atkins dieters usually experience cravings, and that is more apparent during the Pre-Maintenance Phase. Prepare yourself for uncontrollable hunger. This may happen because of reintroducing foods to your diet. Do not forget about the forbidden foods. Steer clear from them. It is also important to listen to your body signals. Give your body sufficient time to adjust before adding another food group back in to your diet.

If some foods upset your body, eliminate them in the meantime. Avoid them for a couple of days. Once your condition improves and you feel like your body's ready to give it another shot then go ahead.

Weight loss plateau is also common so do not be surprised when it feels like you stopped losing when you are not yet on your desired weight. Losing weight may have happened quickly during Induction. However, this phase is meant to be slow and steady. Be patient. Wait it out to know how your body responds. If you really have stopped losing weight and you need to lose a pound or more, cut back 10 grams from your daily net carb allowance.

Rather than a weight loss plateau, some dieters only stumble upon their net carb tolerance, which is ideal for maintaining weight. Make the necessary adjustment and make sure to focus on your goal all the time.

Chapter 7 - The Lifetime Maintenance Phase of the Atkins Diet Program

By the time you reach this phase, you should already be in your desired weight. At this point, there is no more losing. You have reached your weight loss goal. However, your objective changes from losing it to keeping it off permanently.

By being patient slowly transitioning from one phase to another, you have trained yourself to adapt to this new way of eating. Therefore, once you reach this point, it will be much easier to continue the practice. If you can keep at this pace then you are less likely to go back all the way to point A of dieting.

From the Induction phase up to the Pre-maintenance Phase, you have learned moderation and control. At this point, you are familiar with cravings and you are in a better position to control them. As long as you do not let yourself forget what you have learned, you will do just fine.

Substitution is also essential. By being patient enough with the limited food options from phase one up to third, you have learned the value of trading high carb foods from low carb ones. More importantly, you have given yourself a chance to experience the program and allowed yourself to feel the change physically and emotionally. You will lose weight because of the diet program. It is not impossible to keep unwanted weight off by sticking to the rules of the program as well.

What is the goal and purpose of Lifetime Maintenance Phase?

This is the last phase in the Atkins diet program. Rather than looking at it as just another step, it is best to treat it as a permanent change. It is called Lifetime Maintenance after all.

The main reason why many people regain the weight that they have lost is the lack of discipline. The Atkins diet program is meant to change your lifestyle so that you can maintain your desired weight for a lifetime.

What are you allowed to eat during this phase?

There are no additional acceptable foods. Eat as you were eating in the first three phases. Continue reintroducing some of the foods you may have had trouble with reincorporating in your diet in the third phase.

Be patient. Make sure your body is ready to handle these foods to avoid further issues. As long as you are able to maintain your weight goal, you are not in any trouble.

Do not fret when you end up gaining a few pounds in the process of reintroducing foods in your diet. Cut back if you must until you find the most ideal daily net carb allowance for weight maintenance.

If you do regain weight, you can cut back by eliminating any of these foods from your diet.

2 carrots

1 slice of whole-grain bread

1/2 banana

1/2 baked potato

1/2 grapefruit

1/2 sweet potato

1 cup plain yogurt

1 cup watermelon balls

3/4 cup beets

3/4 cup shelled edamame

1/2 cup lentils

1/3 cup chickpeas

1/4 cup brown rice

How to remain in control of your weight?

This is not a phase you will eventually graduate from - unless you want to run the risk of regaining weight. Therefore, it is crucial to stick to your carb tolerance level. This refers to the amount of daily grams of net carbs you can take without gaining additional weight. This is something you will discover from the Pre-Maintenance Phase.

You should also continue allotting around 12 to 15 grams of your daily net carb allowance to foundation vegetables. Continue consuming about 4 to 6 ounces of cooked protein for every meal. If your carb tolerance level allows you to have two servings of fruit per day, do so but never go beyond two servings in one day.

Carbohydrates, fat and protein are all essential for regulating the body's blood sugar response. This is why the Atkins diet program does not completely ban carbs from your diet from the very start. Make sure that your diet has all three not only for successful weight management but more importantly, for your health.

Continue to monitor your weight regularly. Never allow yourself to gain more than 5 pounds. Take immediate action before it comes to that. You can prevent further weight gain by adjusting your carb consumption. It is best to keep counting your carb intake.

Be careful about serving portions. Some foods such as cheese and nuts may trigger you to overeat. To make sure that does not happen, you have to keep measuring. Stick to the assigned portions. Eat nothing more.

Make it a habit to drink plenty of water. Continue to read labels. This is especially critical if you are adding new foods into your diet. As you add new foods, observe how each one affects your body especially when it comes to your cravings and appetite.

Make time for exercise. If you engage in physical activity, adjust your carb consumption accordingly. This is to give your body enough energy.

Finally, you have to know the difference between hunger and habit. When you are overwhelmed with a feeling of hunger, ask yourself whether you are physically or emotionally hungry. Eat for physical hunger and not for the emotional one.

Chapter 8 – Frequently Asked Questions about the Atkins Diet Program

You have already learned a lot about the Atkins diet program from the previous chapters. However, here are a few more tidbits to help set proper expectations before you get started. These are the most common questions and concerns of dieters.

Some dieters say the Atkins diet tends to increase their cholesterol level. Will that happen to me and what can I do to prevent it?

There are dieters who experience an increase in cholesterol especially in the beginning of the program. This is not uncommon. In fact, it usually comes due to weight loss. Cholesterol tends to increase when stored fat is used for energy. However, everything returns to normal in two to three months time.

Increase in HDL cholesterol level may in fact be a good thing. Note that HDL is good cholesterol. It is also important to emphasize that the diet program is not the only reason for the increase in your cholesterol level. Genetic factors are at play here too. In any case, if your cholesterol increases during the program, you can take corresponding supplementation or use essential oils. Do not forget to check with your physician regularly.

Other dieters raise an issue about having bad breath, is it true? Why does it happen and how to avoid it?

As the body burns fat and produce ketones, bad breath may be experienced. This indicates that the diet is actually working. Such problem can be easily treated by consuming dark green leafy vegetables, parsley or sugarless chlorophyll. Drinking a minimum of eight glasses of water a day also proves helpful.

Is constipation an issue?

It will be an issue if you do not hydrate properly. Constipation may happen as your body loses fluids especially during the Induction Phase. This is why it is crucial to replenish lost fluids. It may also be helpful to take supplementary fiber like ground flaxseed, psyllium husks or wheat bran. Eating vegetables, as well as getting exercise is also recommended.

I hear dieters complain about leg cramps. How can I get rid of it in case I experience the same?

In addition to losing fluids, your body may also lose electrolytes that contain potassium, calcium and magnesium. If you do not replenish these lost minerals, you may experience leg cramps. To avoid that, it is advisable to take mineral supplements or simply add salt to your food.

What other side effects do I have to worry about?

Some dieters report headaches as a side effect. One of the most common reasons is caffeine and/ or sugar withdrawal. As you enter the Induction Phase, you will have to give up both. You can take ibuprofen for relief. In other cases, lack of vitamins and dehydration may also result to headaches. Take your vitamin supplements and drink enough water to prevent it from happening.

I'm taking medications. Do I have to stop taking them while on this diet?

If you are taking unnecessary over-the-counter medicines like diuretics, cough syrup, antihistamines, sleep aids, antacids or laxatives, it is best to stop it. There are prescription medications that may also interfere with weight loss. However, before you stop taking them, you must consult with your doctor.

In addition, this diet can cause high blood pressure and lower high blood sugar. If you take oral diabetes medications or insulin, it is necessary to get close supervision during the diet. A few adjustments in your dosage are also necessary. Again, do not make any changes to your medications without consulting your doctor first.

I bought ketosis sticks but they are not changing color. What's wrong? Is the diet not working?

It usually takes two to three days before the body goes to Ketosis. If you are using ketosis sticks for the first two or three days, this could be the reason why the sticks are not changing color. However, if you have tested on the fourth day and there are still no changes, you will have to check on the expiration date of your ketosis sticks. Otherwise, you may be eating more carbs than you should. Check for hidden carbs. Carefully check on how much you are actually consuming.

Conclusion

Thank you again for purchasing this book!

I hope this book was able to help you learn everything that you need to know about losing weight successfully through the Atkins diet program. Laid out here are the details on how you can apply the program from one phase to another. This set of information should allow you to set proper expectations and prepare yourself for the challenges ahead. However, keep in mind that if you follow the rules closely, you can lose weight and keep it off forever.

The next step is to get started. Weigh in. Decide on your weight goal. Get yourself a carb counter. Buy ketosis sticks. Create a chart for monitoring your progress. Write a shopping list. Plan your menu, and always keep your eyes on the prize!

Thank you and good luck!

Printed in Great Britain
by Amazon